LANCHESTER UNIVERSITY

KU-793-717

Lanchester Library

WITHDRAWN

Allergy prevention in infants

Practical advice

B.-M. EXL, Switzerland; A. WALLRAFEN, Germany

NESTLÉ NUTRITION SERVICES

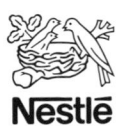

Nestlé

The GERMAN ALLERGY AND ASTHMA ASSOCIATION
(a registered association) is the editor of the German - language
original version of this booklet:
1st edition 1994
2nd revised edition 1995
3rd revised edition 1997
Illustrations/Graphics: © medical vision, Ratingen, Germany.

The editors wish to thank the authors, Dr. B.-M. EXL and
A. WALLRAFEN, as well as the GERMAN ALLERGY AND
ASTHMA ASSOCIATION for their authorizations to publish
this English version.

This guide is a simplified version of the original German edition.

Coventry University

Allergy prevention

Pediatricians are ever more frequently being faced with the problem of "allergies". Some 30 percent of all children up to the age of about 12 are already affected by some hereditary allergic disease! This figure is based not on an estimate but on the findings of many wide-scale investigations. A study conducted in 1989 on almost ten thousand children in Munich, Germany, confirms these findings.

Such chronic diseases cause considerable distress for both children and parents. However, it has been shown that an allergic disease in children with a hereditary predisposition can be influenced from the very first months of life by various environmental factors and more especially by the type of diet they are given. This booklet on allergy prevention is based on these findings.

This booklet is meant to be of assistance to you in consultations with your doctor on precautions to be taken to prevent allergies. The information and practical measures compiled on this subject will help you in assessing your child's risk of developing an allergy and in reducing it, at least to a considerable extent. You should begin taking preventive measures as soon as possible and preferably even before the child is born.

Dear Parents to be!

Allergies and allergic diseases have become an ever more serious health problem and now comprise one of the most frequent forms of childhood disease - and there is a trend to a worsening of both the disease and its severity.

The first manifestation of the so-called "atopic-allergic syndrome" is usually atopic eczema (also known as atopic dermatitis), a skin disease generally involving considerable itching and cutaneous eruptions. It almost always begins during the first year of life, and so it affects primarily infants and small children. In about half of the cases, allergic symptoms disappear by puberty. Yet the frequent itching and other extremely unpleasant cutaneous manifestations are distressing to parents and children alike. Once the main symptoms have abated, about half of the children affected go on to develop hay fever and other respiratory allergies to household pets or house dust mites! This can also be described as "changing patterns" of allergic response.

The aim of this short guide, based on the tried and true principle that "prevention is better than cure", is to help you prevent your child from developing an allergic disease as far as possible during infancy or early childhood. You certainly already know that certain allergies can be inherited. If a child is born into a family with a history of allergies, that alone means that his risk of subsequently developing an allergy is two or even three times higher than that of children who do not have such a predisposition.

The risk of allergy can be determined even before birth. Ask your doctor - your gynecologist or future pediatrician - to check whether your family is to be considered a so-called allergy-prone family. Nowadays, about 35% of all new-borns fall within this group and are at a considerably increased risk for allergy!

Meanwhile, it has been confirmed that a regular low-allergen diet during infancy can reduce the onset of allergic reactions, and particularly atopic eczema, by about half during the first three to five years of life. Providing an allergen-free environment, as far as possible, helps this preventive effect. But even newborns from families with no history of allergies run a 5-15% risk of being allergic. That is why measures for early allergy prevention are increasingly recommended for all new-borns and indeed we have found that they are good for all children!

In this guide, we wish to provide you with a number of important tips on some of the most important allergy-prevention measures to be taken. Background information, tips and nutrition advice should help you to apply everyday individual allergy prevention for your child. For prevention to be as effective as possible, it must begin with your infant's very first feeding. That is why it is important that you start implementing certain recommendations even before your child is born and stick to them as closely as possible.

Unfortunately, no one can guarantee that even if you do faithfully follow all of the preventive measures, your child will not develop some allergy. But several studies have shown that by conscious and consistent prevention, the risk of allergy during the first five years of life can be considerably reduced, at any rate by about one-half.

See your doctor to discuss any questions or uncertainties you may have.

We hope you derive much joy from your child!

Andrea WALLRAFEN
Mönchengladbach, Germany

Dr. Bianca-Maria EXL
St. Légier, Switzerland

Table of contents

① atopic diseases

Atopy - Allergy: What do these terms mean?

Allergens = allergy-triggering substances

By allergy - or also allergic diseases - we mean a hypersensitivity reaction of the body to foreign matter in the environment. This matter, nearly always proteins from pollens, house dust, animal hair (danders), foods and drugs, are called allergens. If an allergic person comes in contact with such allergens - say by eating or breathing or simply contact with the skin - the body reacts with an "excessive" defense reaction. This excessive reaction to matter alien to the body leads to various allergic symptoms. These altered reactions, in which the immune system is always involved, are called allergies.

It is hard to imagine but we now know of over 20,000 such substances which have an allergy-triggering effect!

But a child is never born with an allergy - as it gives its first yell - so to speak. Allergies are acquired over time. This happens mainly through repeated contact with allergens and additional environmental factors - allergen stimuli (or so-called adjuvant factors).

Innate tendency to over-react

If some subjects have an innate tendency to develop a hypersensitivity reaction, which in most persons who subsequently prove to be allergic is the case, we refer to this as an atopic predisposition. So atopies are hypersensitivity reactions which are promoted by a familial predisposition.

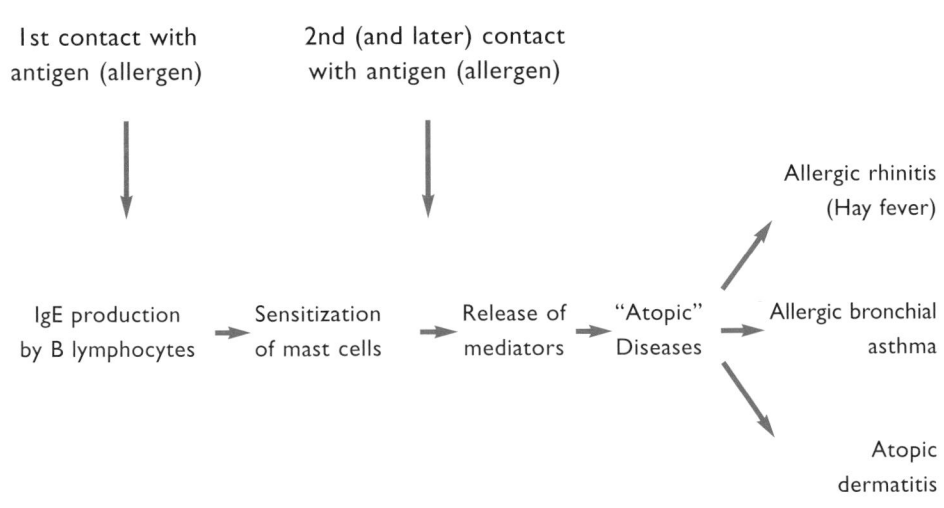

Atopic subjects react to certain antigens (known as allergens) by producing large quantities of specific IgE immunoglobulins*. These IgE are formed by certain white blood cells (B lymphocytes) and bind to the so-called mast cells, thus sensitizing them.

How is an allergic reaction caused?

The next time that such a person comes into contact with the allergy-provoking allergen, mast cell-bound IgE are cross-linked to the allergen, followed by the release of mediators, i.e. histamine, from cellular granules.
Indeed, such mediators cause the multiple symptoms of an "atopic disease".

* Immunoglobulin: a protein with antibody activity found in the blood and other body fluids

Atopic allergic diseases

The following allergic manifestations are referred to as "atopic diseases":

Allergic bronchial asthma
- Frequent coughing with breathing difficulties **but no infection.**
- Clearly audible sounds during inhalation and/or exhalation, known as wheezing.
- Considerable shortness of breath, in some cases after minimal physical exertion.

Allergic rhinitis (Hay fever)
- Seasonal and/or year-round reaction, notably, to pollen, domestic pet hairs (danders) and/or house-dust mites with:
  - Frequent colds and runny noses,
  - Frequent sneezing,
  - In children, frequent nose-rubbing and itchy nose.
- ➢ Yet, **no infection is present.**

Atopic dermatitis (Atopic eczema)
- Itching, red cutaneous eruption:
  - In infants, especially on the cheeks, forehead, chest and arms,
  - In older children and adults, especially on the inner aspect of the forearm and the back of the knees, finger joints and calves.

Food allergies
- Intolerance to certain foods that can manifest as diarrhea, stomach ache, flatulence and/or one or more of the above-mentioned symptoms:
  - Without intestinal infection (viral or bacterial),
  - Without organic gastrointestinal complaints (e.g. lactose intolerance).

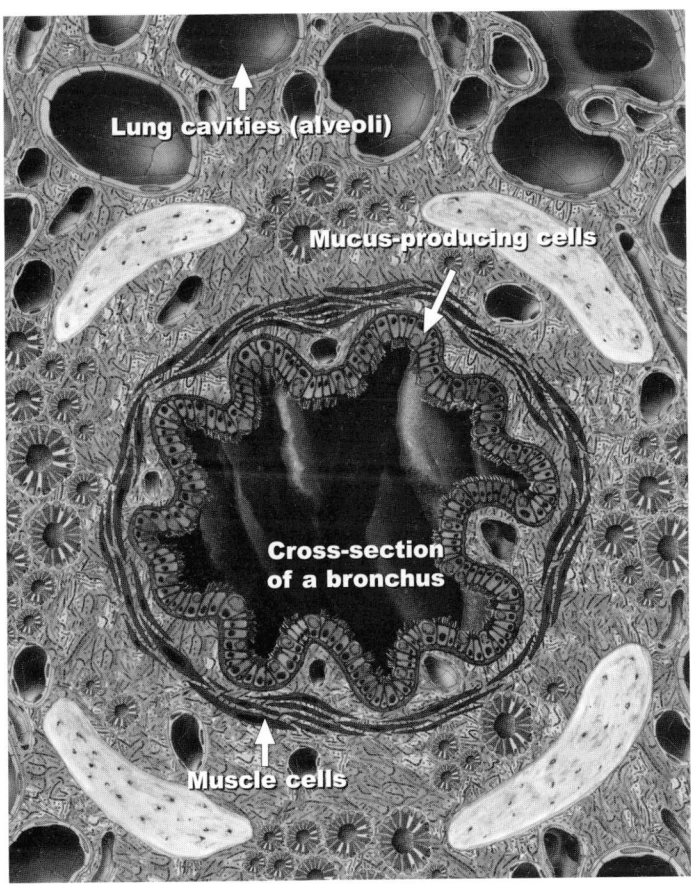

In allergic asthma, an allergen can trigger a cramp-like contraction of the muscle cells surrounding the bronchi, and leads to produce an excess of mucus. This makes breathing extremely difficult and hence the whistling and wheezing sounds related to the labored breathing of asthmatic patients.

Allergic bronchial asthma

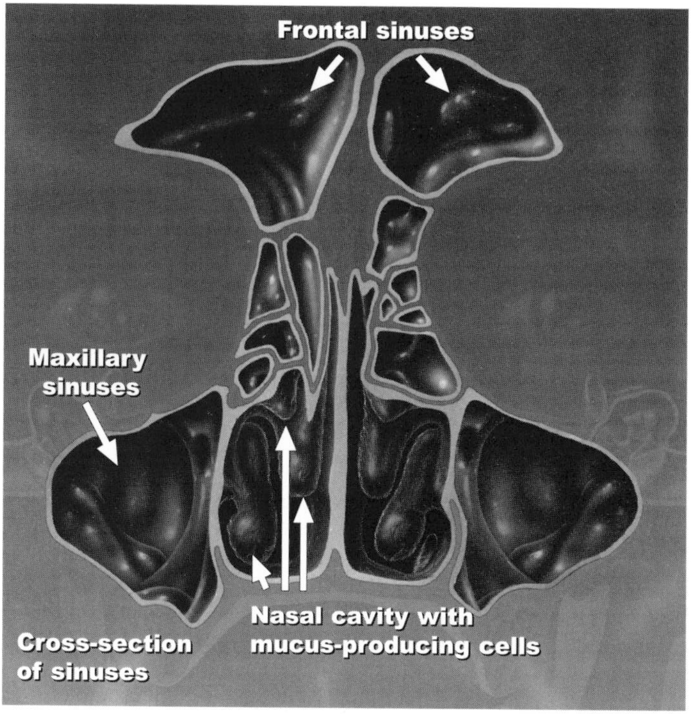
Frontal sinuses
Maxillary sinuses
Nasal cavity with mucus-producing cells
Cross-section of sinuses

Allergic rhinitis

Allergic rhinitis involves "colds with runny nose" without infection. Allergic rhinitis is manifest by runny nose, nasal stuffiness, repeated sneezing, itchy and swollen eyelids can appear all year round or only seasonally when the pollen count is high.

Frequently, not only are the nasal mucosa and the conjunctiva of the eyes affected, but also the mucus-lined sinuses. These mucosa swell, produce increased viscous mucus and cause a build-up of mucus in the sinuses resulting in facial discomfort and headaches.

The skin with its outer horny layer acts as a barrier, protecting the body against the penetration of foreign matter. The underlying (subcutaneous) tissues, in addition, contain the specialized cells of the immune system which also ward off foreign matter and allergens.

In atopic subjects, however, the skin is frequently also the target organ showing the first sign of an allergic disease. So, for example, an itchy, red cutaneous eruption can be caused by an allergy to a particular food or environmental factor and, in infants, this occurs mainly on the cheeks, the forehead, the chest and the arms. In older children, the inner aspect of the forearm and the back of the knee as well as the wrist and calves are affected.

Atopic dermatitis (Atopic eczema)

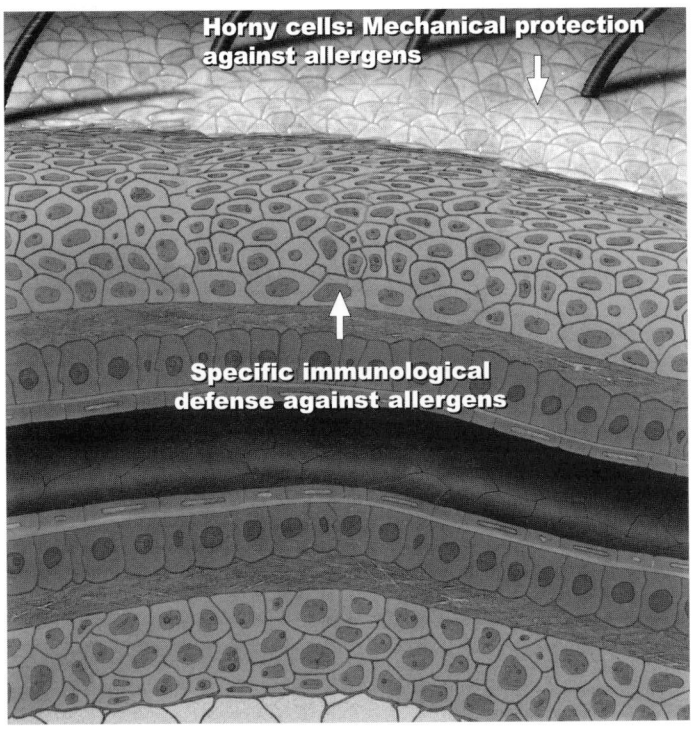

Horny cells: Mechanical protection against allergens

Specific immunological defense against allergens

Atopic diseases do not include:

❶ Contact dermatitis (e.g. nickel allergies)

❷ Sun allergies

❸ Insect bite allergies

❹ Pharmaceutical allergies

❺ Pseudo-allergies:
Histamine hypersensitivity (e.g. to chocolate, red wine, or strawberries)

❻ Hypersensitivity resulting from innate metabolic disturbances

❼ Lactose intolerance

Not all allergies are atopic diseases

These diseases are not determined by heredity. They are either spontaneously acquired allergic reactions (1-4), reactions to symptom-causing substances found directly in foods and which are usually triggered by the allergic reaction itself (5), or by an innate (inherited) metabolic or digestive intolerance to specific substances (6 and 7) such as lactose (milk sugar).

Tobacco smoke "promotes" allergic reactions

If people with a hereditary predisposition for allergies frequently come into contact with allergens and have to cope with aggravating factors such as tobacco smoke, infection, cold, etc., these allergic (or rather atopic) diseases will break out much more frequently and sooner than in people who do not come into contact with tobacco smoke, etc.

Interrelation between inherited and environmental factors in the development of atopic diseases

Hereditary and environmental factors

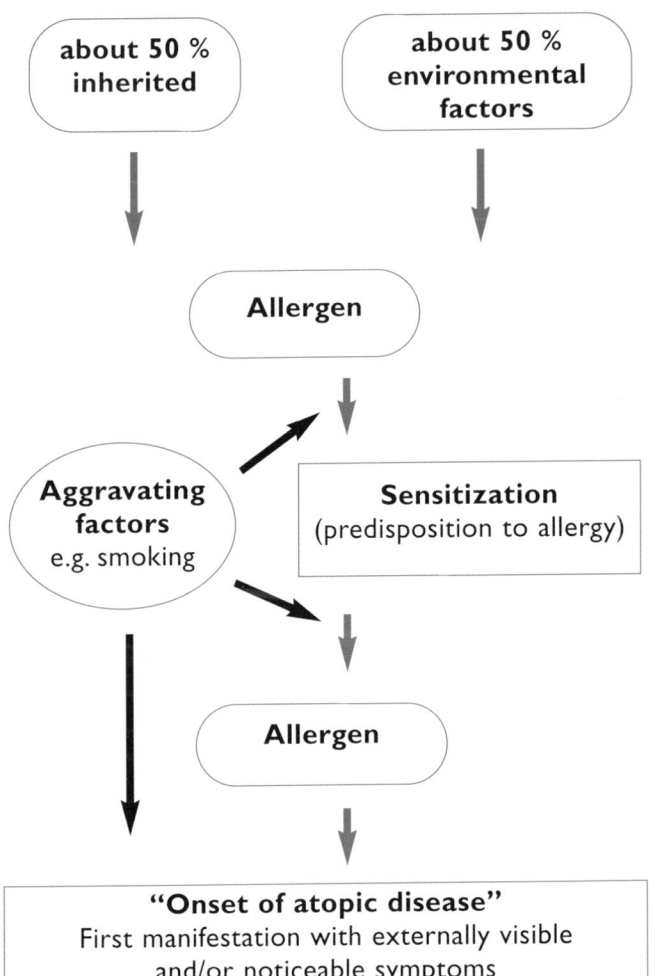

② allergy risk

Can the frequency of allergic disorders in an atopic family be predicted?

The allergy risk in atopic families: up to 80%!

Nowadays, about 25-30% of all children have developed an allergy by the time they reach puberty. In so-called atopic families, the figure is even considerably higher - and can reach 80% if both parents have the same type of allergy.

Do allergies run in the family?

If the frequency of allergic disease among the closest members of the family - father, mother, siblings - is known, then there is also some chance that the subsequent risk of allergy in the newborn can also be predicted. The atopic history of a family must also include those allergies from which the parents suffered during their childhood and which have cleared up in adulthood.

The likelihood of an allergy breaking out in "children at risk" is all the greater, the fewer the preventive measures taken.

Determining the family's risk for allergy

Nowadays, the so-called family history provides the best possible means of determining the risk of allergies in other members of the family. There also other - although less reliable - predictive factors.

The best known method is to measure the total immunoglobulin E (IgE) in the umbilical cord blood of a new-born (umbilical-cord IgE = UC-IgE). Immunoglobulins are proteins present in blood plasma which act as the body's natural defenses, so-called antibodies, against allergens. This method determines whether the baby has already had to contend with allergens in the mother's womb.

Allergy risks and heredity

Risk of allergy in a newborn baby depending on family history:

- Neither parent is allergic → 5-15%
- One parent is allergic → 20-40%
- A sibling is allergic → 25-30%
- Both parents are allergic → 40-60%
- Both parents are allergic with same manifestations → 60-80%

If both parents suffer from the same allergic condition, e.g. atopic dermatitis, the newborn is at highest risk of being allergic.

But even if only one parent or a sibling suffers from an allergy, the risk is markedly higher.

It is now known that there is no absolutely reliable process for clearly estimating the risk of developing an allergy. So, measures which are good for everyone should form the basis of allergy prevention! (See sections on not smoking and special allergen-reduced diets further on).

Does my baby have a high allergy risk?

Determining the allergy risk: as soon as possible

You should ask yourself this question - and get the answer - as soon as possible, that is to say during or even before pregnancy!

Ask your own parents about their childhood

It helps if you fill out the enclosed questionnaire page 21 as soon and carefully as possible to help rapidly clarify the situation. In so doing, it is important to think not only of existing allergies but also those you used to have. This is <u>because</u> atopic diseases can appear in childhood and regress at puberty. That is why it is best to also ask your own parents and those of your partner whether or not they had any allergies during childhood, or you and your partner as kids.

In conducting your "investigation", don't forget that not every sniffle, cough or rash has to be an allergy. (See explanations on pages 8-14).

Discuss the questionnaire with the doctor

In any event, it is advisable for you to discuss the questionnaire with your family doctor, pediatrician, gynecologist, or an allergy specialist. With the help of this information, you and the respective specialist doctor can soon provide a fairly precise prediction of your child's risk for allergy.

EVALUATING THE FAMILY QUESTIONNAIRE

Even one "yes" means increased risk

Even one "yes" reply on the questionnaire, indicating that some member of your family has an allergic predisposition considerably increases the allergy risk for your baby. <u>However</u>, even babies whose families have no history of allergies may themselves run a risk of some 5 to 15% of subsequently having an allergy.

With the help of the table on page 19 you can determine your child's exact risk as a percentage.

Family questionnaire for estimating the allergy risk of a newborn

Type of allergy* (see pp.8-14)	No family member affected	Mother	Father	Siblings
Atopic dermatitis Atopic eczema, Endogenous eczema				
Allergic bronchial asthma Allergic bronchitis				
Allergic rhinitis Allergic (runny) "cold" e.g. hay-fever, Year-round allergic "cold"				
Food allergy (not simple intolerance)				

* always without infection

(3) practical recommendations

Can the first manifestation of an allergy be prevented, diminished or delayed?

By taking preventive measures you can actually ensure during the first years of life that the so-called first manifestation of an allergy does not develop at all or is at least delayed. The findings of many wide-scale investigations agree in that this is not just wishful thinking.

In about half of all children with a considerably exacerbated risk of allergy, the onset of an allergy in the first three to five years of life can be prevented. This is particularly so for atopic dermatitis (atopic eczema) which in about 90% of all cases is the first manifestation of all types of allergies.

50% fewer allergies in the first three to five years

Although one hundred percent protection is not possible, much can however be done with relatively simple and moreover low-cost preventive measures that can be in addition recommended for all children - far more indeed, than anyone had originally dared to hope.

Total protection is not possible

The following table gives you some idea of existing effective preventive measures. Then, in subsequent chapters, each of these measures will be presented and explained in detail. You should refer to it often so that it may serve as a practical reminder and help you in the daily implementation of your allergy-prevention measures.

Preventive measures: A summary to keep in mind

Practical recommendations for preventing allergies in newborns in allergy-prone families

Summary from the opinion issued by the EU Scientific Committee on Food (SCF, 1991), the European Society for Pediatric Gastroenterology, Hepatology and Nutrition (ESPGHAN, 1993), the Nutritional Commission of the German Pediatric Society (1996), and the publications by Zeiger (1990, 1995), Koletzko and Schmidt (1991), Wahn (1992), Chandra (1997), Zeiger (1995), as well as Vandenplas (1995, 1998).

Basic principles	Practical measures
I Recognizing the risks of allergies	• Recording the **family allergy history** with the special family history questionnaire and yours doctor's help

II Dietary guidelines (Principles to be recommended for all newborns)

(a) Infant feeding	• If at all possible, **exclusively breastfeed your baby for the first 4-6 months**. Do not give any supplementary conventional cow's milk or soybean based formula even and especially not in the maternity clinic. • If it is not possible to solely breastfeed your infant, only well-tested* **low-allergen, i.e. hypoallergenic, infant formula** should be given (so called H.A. formula). • **Weaning foods should not be given too early, i.e. before the end of the 4th, or better still, the 6th month**. Avoid strongly allergenic foods for the entire first year (see list on page 57). • After beginning the introduction of weaning foods, broaden the diet by adding just one new food per week.
(b) Mother's diet during pregnancy and breastfeeding	• **No special diet during pregnancy and breastfeeding**. Just a well-balanced, high-vitamin diet. • If the mother herself has a (food-) allergy, possibly reduce known food allergens during the breastfeeding period. ** • Take 1 gr of calcium per day as a nutritional supplement, if the mother is on a special diet.
	Important: A mother's strict diet should be observed only under the supervision of a doctor and a dietitian.

* Hypoallergenic infant formulas tested according to the recommendations of the European Society for Pediatric Gastroenterology, Hepatology and Nutrition (ESPGHAN) and complying with the EC Infant Formula Directive (edition of 16.2.96). Nestlé H.A. formulas as Nan H.A., Nidina H.A., Nativa H.A., Nidal H.A., Guigoz H.A., Good Start, Aletemil H.A. and Beba H.A. meet these European guidelines.

** See page 39 for major food allergens. Important note only if you have yourself a severe food allergy: watch the list of ingredients as these foods are often unsuspectedly included!

III Negative environmental factors

Smoking
- Try to keep the environment smoke-free both before and after the birth of your child.

Animal hairs
- Avoid early contact with animal hairs (danders): household pets, horse-hair mattresses, duvets, fluffy toys, sheepskins, camel-hair blankets, etc. as well as clothing made from such substances.
- It is recommended that cotton clothing be washed first before wearing.

House dust mites
Measures that make it harder for house dust mites to survive:
- Cool dry rooms.
- Regular airing of the <u>whole</u> appartment or house, but not in the morning.
- Mattress covers that mites cannot penetrate or wash bed linen at 90°C degrees.
- Avoid "dust-traps" such as heavy curtains, potted plants, upholstered furniture, open shelves.
- Wet cleanable floor or short-pile carpets or fitted carpets:
    - Do not use the vacuum cleaner in your child's presence,
    - Use air filters and vacuum cleaners with filters of certified performance.

Mildew
- Regularly maintain air-conditioning and air-humidifying equipment as these can easily be attacked by mildew.
- Air the house regularly (see house dust mites).
- Avoid potted plants in garden mould. Hydroculture is better.
- Immediately remove damp patches.

Pollen
- Avoid any early contact with flowers, grass, hazelnut blossom, wheat or birch pollen.
- Keep windows closed from the early morning when the pollen count is high.
- Do not undress in the bedroom.

IV Other factors
- Do not have your infant's and young children's ears pierced. Danger of nickel allergy!
- Try to avoid frequent contact with other children during the first six months to prevent early infection.
- Keep away from adults with colds as certain infections facilitate the development of allergies.
- Do not use any baby-care products containing milk protein.
- Do not use highly-perfumed baby-care products.

Proper nutrition is of the utmost importance in preventing allergies. During breastfeeding, mothers with (food-) allergies themselves most probably remove from their shopping lists any foods which they know contain aggressive food allergens anyway (see page 39).

When gradually introducing supplementary foods into the baby's diet, foods known to be powerfully allergenic should generally be avoided. However, it is important that both mother and child receive a well-balanced diet rich in vitamins and minerals during pregnancy, breastfeeding and infancy.

Especially when the mother is on a diet (avoiding certain foods), she should always seek good nutritional advice in order to ensure well-balanced nutrition. For example, if she is avoiding cow's milk, she should drink mineral water rich in calcium and take about 1 g of supplementary calcium (in effervescent tablets) each day.

④ pregnancy

What about prenatal allergy prevention?

A diet is not necessary!

There is no reason to follow a specific diet during pregnancy. This recommendation is based on the findings of several studies where no diet was shown to produce any positive effect.

Even though you may find it a bit difficult, for your baby's sake you should avoid smoking and also taking alcoholic drinks in general.
Stimulants such as alcohol certainly have little to do with allergy prevention but they do harm your child.

Food rich in vitamins and minerals

Make sure that your menu is as varied as possible and contains plenty of fresh fruit and vegetables. This will help meet your increased vitamin and mineral requirements during pregnancy.

TIPS FOR EQUIPPING THE FUTURE NURSERY

Parquet or linoleum rather than fitted carpets

Equip the nursery in such a way as to keep it as free as possible of materials of animal origin. This, for example, concerns the bed (no horsehair mattress!), the rest of the furnishings and also, of course, the floor where preference should be given to short-pile carpets, parquet or vinyl flooring rather than high-pile carpets.

Under-floor heating also has a beneficial effect on the atmosphere in the room as it keeps the floor dry, making it considerably harder for mites to survive!

Protection from house dust mites

Carpets and fitted carpets can be cleaned with so-called acaricide products (which kill mites). The cleaning should, however, not be undertaken by persons who are themselves allergic.

Mattresses which are more than 8 years old should, in all cases, be replaced by new mattresses. Of recent years, it has been possible to find special mite-resistant or mite-proof mattress covers on the market. These drastically reduce the concentrations of mites to which the person is exposed and help alleviate symptoms in persons already affected. The mattresses are enclosed in these covers which can also be washed or cleaned and the mites already in the mattress can no longer get out.

Mattress covers, known as "fitted covers" and bed linen that can be boiled

Eiderdowns and pillowcases should be washable at 95°C. If they are not washable at that temperature, they must be washed for at least 1 hour at 60°C in order to kill off the mites. Mite-proof bed linen can now be found in the appropriate specialized linen shops.

Upholstered furniture must also be cleaned regularly. However, leather furniture does not harbor mites.

Leather upholstery instead of fabrics

AND ONE MORE TIP: Fluffy toys can be rid of their mites after a few hours in the deep freezer.

Fluffies in the freezer

FURTHER TIPS AGAINST MILDEW

Proper ventilation prevents the formation of mildew:

- Air rooms only actively, when a room is actually being used.

- Adapt airing time to weather conditions, that is, the colder it is outside, the shorter the airing time.

- Always air with the window wide open. In Winter, every two hours for about four minutes.

AND FINALLY SOME COMMENTS ON HOUSEHOLD PETS

Keep household pets away from baby for the first year!

Wait until your child is at least one year old before acquiring a household pet.

If, however, you already have a cat or dog or any other furry pet, keep it at a "distance" from your child until the child is one year old. Even though it may be difficult, neither your baby nor, where possible, yourself should have any close contact with the household pet. This is so if only because of the danger of contamination or infection especially from cats not confined to the house. The allergizing rate is particularly high with real "pet mice" and "pet rats"!

As for animals

Prepare an animal-hair-free room for your child which is absolutely "off-limits" to your household pet. It actually also makes sense regularly to wipe your pet down with a damp cloth after combing its coat.

⑤ maternity clinic

How should the infant be fed during the first days of its life?

Breast milk protein is not allergenic

The ideal nutritional protein for your baby is the protein in mother's milk. Your baby's body produces no allergic reaction to this protein because it recognizes it as derived from its own body. However, some foreign proteins eaten by the mother may pass into breast milk and are thought to normally induce oral tolerance to those proteins. Breastfeeding remains therefore the best way to protect your baby from developing allergies.

Provide energy without protein allergens for the first three days after birth

It is perfectly normal that, during the first few days after delivery, very little milk is formed. This milk precursor, called "colostrum", is particularly valuable as it is rich in factors that protect the new-born from infection. Heavy milk production generally starts between the 3rd and the 6th days postpartum. In order to make up the lack of milk or necessary energy during the first two of three days after birth and until the milk begins to flow, the maternity nurses will probably give your baby maltodextrin solutions which are the most suitable supplements as they provide energy but no protein.

Absolutely refuse to let your child be given cow's milk or soy-based infant formula supplements:
Some maternity wards tend to give this, especially at night.
If any supplements are required, only hypoallergenic infant formulas should be used.

There are cases in which the baby may require supplementary feeding earlier:

- If the baby loses more than 5% of its birth weight.
- If it was already underweight at birth.

Rule of thumb for supplementary feeding:

A new-born child should receive such supplementary feeding from the third or at latest the fourth day if the mother's milk does not yet suffice.

If your baby needs supplementary feeding, ensure that he or she receives a hypoallergenic, i.e. low-allergen infant formula. Such infant formula is often referred to by the abbreviation "H.A.". The exact product name used may vary depending on country, and not all "H.A." formulas meet the necessary requirements.

Hypoallergenic infant formula

When such H.A. formula is manufactured the protein is processed in such a way so what it is split into smaller components which do not induce any more sensitizations to this protein.

Nourishing and low in allergens

And one more important point:

Make sure that whatever happens, use only a hypoallergenic formula that has been tested and approved in accordance with the requirements of the scientific committees of the SCF* and ESPGHAN** (see page 26).

Furthermore, the formula should meet the nutritional requirements set up by local legislation or by international bodies, such as the EU Directive for starter infant formulas*** in Europe, the Infant Formula Act in United States, Codex standard for infant formulas on a worldwide basis.

*SCF= EU Scientific Committee on Food.

**ESPGHAN = European Society of Pediatric Gastroenterology, Hepatology and Nutrition.

***The European Directive on Infant and Follow-up Formulas amended on 16.2.1996.
The amendment to the European Directive includes low-allergen (hypoallergenic) infant formula for allergy prevention. These have to be tested for suitability in clinical trials.

⑥ breastfeeding

Is there a special diet for the mother during breastfeeding?

Human milk: the best nourishment for your child!

Human milk is the best nourishment for your child! This is particularly true of allergy prevention. Not only is human milk hypoallergenic but it also contains immune factors that will help your child to build up his immune system at an early age. By giving only breast milk for four to six months without any additional so-called supplements, you are providing the best possible protection of your baby against any possible allergy. However, by the sixth month at the latest you will have to start giving supplements, as human milk no longer provides sufficient nourishment.

Diet during breastfeeding?

There has been and continues to be considerable discussion as to whether there is any point in following a special diet during breastfeeding. We now have the results of a study which indicates that breastfed children from allergy-prone families have even less eczema if the mother does not follow a specific diet. This study shows that the few allergens that are in breast milk induce tolerance in the baby and prepare the child for normal foods later on which contain many allergens.

Human milk: the best protection against allergies!

The cause of hypersensitive reactions in breastfed infants usually lies in an unintentional deviation from preventive dietary measures for the child. Known examples of this are biscuits made with milk or bath and shampoo products that contain milk or egg white. Even contamination by food on the fingers or in house dust contain many more allergens than human milk alone! So, to say it clearly once more, even without a diet, human milk is the best way to protect your child against allergies.

Should you, despite this, and because of a food-allergy yourself, decide to go on a particular diet, do not under any circumstances try to do it alone but consult your doctor and a specialised dietitian. This is the only way you can be really sure of doing everything necessary to ensure that you have a well-balanced, nourishing diet - unless, of course, you yourself suffer from some food allergy and have become a specialist in the matter.

Do not diet without your doctor's advice!

Foods which should be taboo in a low-allergen mother's diet:

- Fish
- Eggs
- Wheat
- Citrus fruits
- Nuts, especially peanuts and hazelnuts
- Soy and soy products
- Celery

Milk and milk products should be consumed in moderate quantities (less than 250 ml per day).

IMPORTANT:

❶ If you do not suffer from a food allergy yourself, it generally suffices if you refrain from "knowingly" using these products, that is to say, if you remove them from your shopping list. It is no great tragedy if one or another of these foods crops up as a so-called latent ingredient in some ready-made product that you may eat.

Make sure you get extra calcium!

❷ If you go for a low-allergen diet and give up milk and dairy products you are going to lack the most important source of the mineral calcium which is particularly necessary during breastfeeding. You should, therefore, take your daily requirement of one gram of calcium per day in the form of effervescent tablets which are also available in the form of a food supplement and drink a lot of calcium containing mineral water. Your doctor will certainly be pleased to advise on how you can ensure that you receive sufficient calcium.

Eat fresh fruit and vegetables!

❸ Other than that you will be providing both yourself and your child with proper nutrition by eating a wide range of fresh fruit (not citrus) and vegetables.

Cookbooks for a low-allergen diet

A very useful source of assistance is found in special cookbooks in which you will find all there is to know and many important tips and suggestions about how to follow a strict or even an easy-going low-allergy diet.

Other questions on allergy prevention during pregnancy, breastfeeding or feeding infant formulas:

A little reminder when you see your doctor or dietitian

....

....

....

....

....

....

....

....

....

....

Special Comments:

....

....

....

....

....

$\textcircled{7}$ adapting feeds

What to do if the mother's milk does not suffice?

Drink liquids and sleep enough

Certain situations such as stress or physical fatigue often result in a temporary drop in breast milk supply. Do not let this upset or alarm you. Try to stay calm, drink plenty of liquids and get enough sleep - as far as your baby will let you! Above all, breast feed him as often as possible. You will see that before long your milk will again fully suffice.

Hypoallergenic "H.A. formula": equivalent allergy prevention

If, during this temporary phase, you do have to provide supplementary feeding or if despite all your efforts your milk really doesn't suffice, then give your baby one of the described hypoallergenic or low-allergen infant formulas. These will protect your child against allergies just as well as would mother's milk (see pages 26, 34-36 and 45).

Many tests concur in showing that children from allergy-prone families, fed with conventional cow's milk or soy based infant formulas, were twice as likely to react with an allergy or intolerance than were infants that had been fed human milk or a hypoallergenic infant formula.

Simple to prepare

The preparation of hypoallergenic formula is as easy as that of classical infant formulas. Simply mix the powder with previously boiled water in accordance with the instructions. How much you give the baby will, exactly as with human milk, depend solely on your baby's requirements. So you can perfectly well give the baby as much as he wants!

But for consistent allergy prevention, you should also pay attention to give your baby only a hypoallergenic formula as exclusive diet throughout the first four to six months. So do not give your baby any additional "extras". This applies regardless of whether you continue to breastfeed or shift completely to an H.A. formula.

No "extras"!

In Europe and in other parts of the world the following clinically tested Nestlé hypoallergenic infant formulas comply with the international guidelines:
- Aletemil H.A.
- Beba H.A.
- Guigoz H.A.
- Good Start
- Nan H.A.
- Nativa H.A.
- Nidal H.A.
- Nidina H.A.

Finally, here is just one more bit of advice. The special composition of hypoallergenic infant formula could result in your baby's stools having a color similar to how they were during breastfeeding, that is to say greenish in color. Do not let that worry you as it is perfectly normal when feeding on this formula. The stools are also softer, as when feeding on human milk.

Don't worry about stool color!

Soft stools are desirable

45

⑧ feeding problems

Parents often lack confidence, especially with the first child: "What should I do if my baby isn't really satisfied, if he has gas or suddenly has diarrhea?"
Basically, you should always talk to your doctor before changing the formula. But here are some tips and advice on the most frequent problems that crop up in infants, and mainly the problems are not related to the formula.

In order to avoid mistakes and worry when changing the diet you should as a matter of principle discuss any of these changes with your doctor:

Ask your doctor!

- The first administration of supplementary H.A. formula during breastfeeding if the mother's milk does not suffice.
- Switching to H.A. formula when you wish to stop breast-feeding.
- Changing from H.A. formula to some other infant formula.
- Introducing supplementary feeding especially using products containing cow's milk.

What to do if the baby suffers from bloating and gas?

Intestinal gas is a frequent problem with young infants. In most cases this unpleasant side effect has nothing to do with the formula given, as even breastfed infants are not spared! The reason for this is often the air that the baby swallows when drinking or crying. A few simple prevention measures can help to avoid or reduce the problem.

Important tips that can help with "excess gas"

- Always try to feed your baby in a "relaxed atmosphere".

- Remember to "burp" the baby during or after feeding so that the air can escape from his stomach.

- Help your baby to release gas by placing him on your shoulder and patting him on the back while "strolling around", gently stroking and soothing him.

- The nipple is also important: It should always be soft and smooth and have the right size hole so that the contents of the bottle drips out slowly when it is tilted.

Massaging, "burping" and the right nipple...

- The baby does not like milk froth so you are better off leaving that in the bottle!

- Carefully massage your baby's tummy in a clockwise direction.

- Do gymnastics with your baby, carefully press his legs against his stomach a number of times.

But in any event, talk to your pediatrician if your baby frequently suffers from gas. This is especially true if this problem is persistent and of long duration and is not relieved by the recommendations given above.

Help! my baby has the "runs"! (diarrhea)

An electrolyte solution will do the trick

If your baby has diarrhea, it will normally be quite enough for you to give him an electrolyte solution (oral rehydration solution) which can be recommended and prescribed by your doctor.

If you are breastfeeding, you need do nothing other than administer the electrolyte solution and continue breastfeeding. As a rule, the diarrhea will then disappear of its own accord. If you are using an H.A. formula, you can continue to use it as well.

But, please always ask your doctor's advice!

Be careful with special therapeutic formulas

If your baby's diarrhea is severe or lasts so long that specific antidiarrheal medicinal formula is needed, **it too must be hypoallergenic.**

Attention:

Very often, so-called "special therapeutic" do not contain hypoallergenic proteins, so it is advisable that you consult your doctor about an antidiarrhea diet before making your choice.

What do you do if your baby is not satisfied?

What do you do if, before the age of six months, your baby is no longer satisfied with breast milk and/or H.A. formula?

Firstly, try to feed the baby more often and, if possible, do without supplementary feeding.

You may also switch to a hypoallergenic H.A. follow-up formula such as Nestlé Nan H.A.2. Only if these are no longer sufficient, should you start with introduction of a cereal pap in your baby's diet.

From the stand point of allergy prevention, rice is relatively unproblematic as it is considered only mildly allergenic. Hence, even in cases of food allergies, rice is used as a component of what is known as an "elimination diet". But, be careful, this is not the case in Asian countries, where rice allergies are rather frequent!

Low-allergen supplements

If you do use rice pap, it should however contain no dried milk and should be prepared with H.A. formula - but never use fresh milk!

---

⑨ from six months on

Can allergy prevention with weaning foods be continued?

*"Positive list":
help with plan-
ning a diet.*
The time has now come to diversify your baby's diet by adding a maximum of one new type of supplementary food per week (see examples on pages 55-56). In this way you will rapidly recognize and also immediately be able to remove any food to which the baby is intolerant. All you need to do is simply stop giving that food.

Compile a sort of "positive list" containing all the foods that your baby tolerates well. This list will then help to plan your child's diet in a varied and uncomplicated fashion.

*Look out for prod-
ucts low in
nitrates and
harmful sub-
stances*
To be sure, when composing your child's diet, you should stick to foods known to be safe for babies and low in harmful substances such as nitrates. It is advisable that you give preference to industrial weaning foods (either deshydrated cereals products or baby foods in jars) which are produced under the strict provisions of dietary legislation and are subjected to additional checks.

Obviously, you can prepare the supplementary food yourself. However, if you do, don't forget to make certain that you obtain starting ingredients which are low in pesticides and nitrates!

We would recommend that as you build up supplementary feeding you try, as far as possible, to use simple products (products comprising only one ingredient such as apples). A meal should contain no more than three simple ingredients, (e.g. chicken, carrots and potatoes).

One-component and simply-combined product

When introducing supplementary feeding, you must always pay attention to make certain that, up to your child's first birthday, you avoid all foods that are known to be particularly likely to cause allergies (see list on page 57).

To give you a clearer idea of the transition phase coming up, we have provided below a plan which you can use as an example. But in all cases you should discuss the timing and composition of supplementary feeding with your pediatrician.

How and when to add supplements: ask your doctor!

EXAMPLES:

❶ You can, for example, begin with a carrot product. Start with a few spoonfuls and gradually increase the amount.

❷ If your baby tolerates the carrots well you can, during the following week, add potatoes to the carrots. You could, of course, also start with some fruit such as, for example, "baby apple" or "baby pear" and, by the second week, you could perfectly well try a two-fruit compote such as, for example, bananas with apple.

Giving ready-made supplements

❸ If that, too, is well tolerated then, after about four weeks, your baby can certainly have a first complete meal. You can use the existing range of simply composed single baby products and baby menus such as, for example:

- Baby carrots
- Baby apples
- Carrots with potatoes and chicken.

Prepare cereal paps with follow-up milk During the baby's second half of the first year, pediatricians recommend using follow-up formulas instead of fresh milk. So, to prepare cereal paps replace fresh milk by follow-up formula, and add the appropriate amount of baby cereal.

Hypoallergenic follow-up formula If you wish to be quite sure and not give your child any unaltered milk protein for the first full year, you could use hypoallergenic H.A. follow-up formula instead of normal follow-up milk.

And once again:

Please, always remember to discuss each new step with your pediatrician. Also inform him immediately if your baby shows any intolerance so that the cause can be determined as quickly as possible!

Feeding recommendations for the first year of your child's life

From the first to the fourth month
For the first four to six months of your child's life, feed baby exclusively:
- Breast milk
- and/or a clinically tested hypoallergenic infant formula (H.A. formula) (see page 45).

From the fifth to the seventh month
Begin at the earliest at the start of the fifth month-or even better after the sixth month by slowly and carefully adding supplementary foods.

In so doing, please observe the following:
- Breast milk and/or hypoallergenic infant follow-up formula
- No supplementary food containing milk
- No eggs No citrus fruits
  No fish No wheat products
  No soy bean products No tomatoes or celery
  No nuts or peanuts No chocolate
- Add only one new additional food per week

Mix instant infant cereal powder with hypoallergenic infant follow-up formula instead of fresh milk in the usual way.

From the seventh to the twelfth month
By the seventh month, you can slowly expand supplementary feeding but if possible:
- No fresh milk (instead of which you should use follow-up formulas or if necessary hypoallergenic follow-up formulas)
- No eggs
- No nuts or peanuts
- No fish
- No soybean products
- No chocolate or cocoa
- No citrus fruits
- No peas
- No tomatoes or celery

After baby's first birthday
You may gradually switch to more liberal feeding, i.e. light, low-salt adult food.

Please be careful to introduce each new food individually and at 2 to 3 day intervals in order to see if and how your child tolerates it!

⑩ allergic reaction

What to do if excessive allergic reactions occur despite prevention?

Prevention is no guarantee!

Even if you take all the preventive measures, no one, unfortunately, can guarantee that an allergic disorder will never appear.

Should you notice any adverse reaction in your child (e.g. itchy cutaneous eruption, gastrointestinal disorders, inflammation of the conjunctive tissues or breathing problems, in each case without any bacterial or viral infection, see pages 8-14), this may indicate an allergy, and so please immediately consult your pediatrician. Only in this way can you be sure of a proper diagnosis and more especially the appropriate treatment.

"Allergy diary" helps with the diagnosis

An "allergy diary" can be helpful and also greatly facilitate your doctor's job. In this "diary", you should consistently list all foods used and each factor that could in any way influence your child's health. Here you should, for example, also think of the above-mentioned baby-care products as well as the clothes and toys with which your child comes in contact - not forgetting house pets and materials in the bedroom.

There are different cookbooks that can give you practical tips for keeping to a strict elimination diet but also for diets that can help seek out the cause of an allergy and even recipes for low-irritant supplementary feeding for infants up to one year of age.

My notes and observations of my child's food intolerance:

Date	Food	Allergic reaction
....	....	....
....	....	....
....	....	....
....	....	....
....	....	....
....	....	....
....	....	....
....	....	....
....	....	....
....	....	....
....	....	....
....	....	....
....	....	....

Special Comments:

....

....

....

....

....

Important notice

The World Health Organisation (WHO*) has recommended that pregnant women and new mothers be informed of the benefits and superiority of breastfeeding - in particular the fact that breast-milk provides the best nutrition and protection from illness for babies.

Mothers should be given guidance on the preparation for, initiation and maintenance of lactation, with special emphasis on the importance of a well-balanced diet both during pregnancy and after delivery. Unnecessary introduction of partial bottle-feeding or other foods and drinks should be discouraged since it will have a negative effect on breastfeeding. Similarly, mothers should be warned of the difficulty of reversing a decision not to breastfeed.

Before advising a mother to use an infant formula, she should be advised of the social and financial implications of her decision. If a baby is exclusively bottle-fed, more than one can (450 g) per week will be needed, so the family circumstances and costs should be kept in mind. Mothers should be reminded that breast-milk is not only the best, but also the most economical, convenient and bacteriologically safe food for babies.

If a decision to use an infant formula is taken, it is important to give instructions on correct preparation methods, emphasizing that unboiled water, unsterilized bottles or incorrect dilution can all lead to illness.

* See: International Code of Marketing of Breast Milk Substitutes, adopted by the World Health Assembly in Resolution WHA 34.22, May 1981.

© 1998, Nestec S.A., CH-1800 Vevey, Switzerland.
Printed in Switzerland.

All rights reserved. No part of this publication may be reproduced,
recorded or transmitted in any form and by any medium whatsoever
(electronic, mechanical, photocopying, recording or other) without the
written permission of the publisher.

The material contained in this publication was submitted as previously
unpublished material, except where credit is given to a source of part
of the material illustrated.

Nestec S.A. has taken great care to check the accuracy of the information contained in this publication. Nevertheless, Nestec S.A. cannot
be held responsible for any errors or omissions, or for any conse-
quences arising from the use of the information it contains. With particular regard to drugs, the reader must refer to the manufacturer's
recommendations for the dosage, especially if the reader is not in the
habit of using the product to be administered or prescribed, or if he
has not used it for some time.

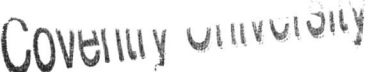